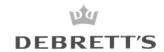

DEBRETT'S

MEN'S STYLE

DEBRETT'S POCKET BOOKS

DEBRETT'S POCKET BOOKS

MEN'S STYLE

Published by Debrett's Limited
18–20 Hill Rise
Richmond
Surrey TW10 6UA

www.debretts.com

Text Jo Bryant

Design Karen Wilks

Editorial Jo Bryant, Liz Wyse

ISBN 9781870520003

Printed and bound by Butler Tanner & Dennis Ltd,
Frome and London

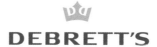

MEN'S STYLE

DEBRETT'S POCKET BOOKS

CONTENTS

"A man should look as if
he had bought his clothes
with intelligence, put them
on with care, and then
forgotten all about them."
Hardy Amies

~ It's more than just clothes ~

WHAT IS STYLE?

STYLE HAS NEVER BEEN ABOUT WHAT YOU WEAR. At least not entirely. Style is an attitude, it is a confidence, a bearing, poise and personality. The most stylish gentleman is not the man dripping in labels, but the man who can turn heads simply because of who he is and how he holds himself. The best way to be stylish is simply to be comfortable in yourself, hold your head high and own every room into which you walk.

HOW TO BE STYLISH

☛ **Be confident:** your suit might be perfectly tailored, but your attitude within it is what counts. ☛ *Care about how you look – but don't care too much: stay sharp, but constant readjustments display vanity not style.* ☛ **Wear clothes that fit:** it may sound silly, but it's amazing how often it's forgotten. ☛ *Be yourself: it's harder to make someone else's look work better than your own.* ☛ **When in doubt, go classic:** some trends come and go and others don't – there is a reason. ☛ *Put your back into it: by which, we mean, stand up straight. It makes you look bigger, stronger and more confident.* ☛ **Experiment:** sometimes it pays to be adventurous.

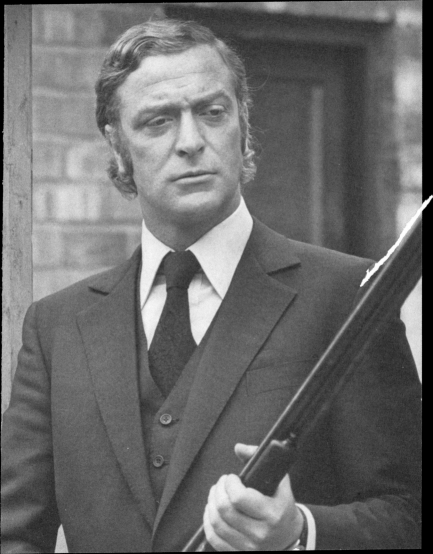

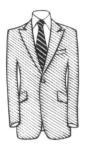 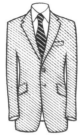 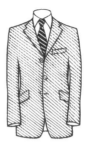 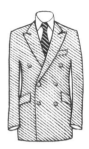

SUIT BASICS

HOW TO WEAR A SUIT

NEVER THINK OF YOUR SUIT AS A UNIFORM – it should be designed to make you look impressive and be worn with individual flair. A suit should improve your posture as it will give you a structure, so stand tall but not to attention – you should try to look at ease. When you sit down in a suit, pull your trousers up at the top of the knees to lessen any strain. You should also unbutton your coat, especially if wearing a double-breasted suit. If you're required to wear a suit for work, your wardrobe should boast three suits of varying colours.

DOUBLE-BREASTED SUITS

The shape of the coat accentuates the chest, so opt for a sleek (rather than boxy) fit. This is a good choice for slim, athletic men.

THREE-BUTTON SUITS

Less versatile than other styles and best worn by tall men. Try to only do up the middle button; never do up the lowest button.

TWO-BUTTON SUITS

A flattering and versatile silhouette; a good all-rounder for most builds. The lower button should remain undone.

ONE-BUTTON SUITS

Simple and stylish, the sleek fit and single button creates smooth, clean lines. Ideal for slim and shorter men. Wear buttoned-up.

PATTERNS

Vertical stripes add height, and the bigger you are, the wider the stripe you can wear. Checks are less formal but they are for the brave and bold; a good alternative is a herringbone. If you are wary of patterns, remember that a classic plain suit will never look wrong.

TEXTURE

Enhance a plain suit by adding a woven texture. A twill weave will give your suit a nicely cut finish with a slight sheen; a coarser fabric will create a matt finish.

LININGS

Suit linings are a chance to add a dash of flair to your suit. Always choose a lining that will work with the colour of the shirts you most often wear with your suit.

SAVILE ROW STYLE

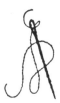
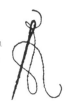

For centuries, Savile Row has been the home of British tailoring, offering generations of experience and knowledge. Here you will find a uniquely bespoke service, offering some of the highest levels of tailoring craftsmanship in the world. A Savile Row suit is like no other; cared for correctly, it will last for decades.

SUIT TRADITIONS

SECRET SIGNALS

A bespoke traditional Savile Row suit will feature a few details that identify its heritage. These include a hand-sewn, pearl stitch buttonhole on the right lapel, above the breast pocket, and a named, dated label stitched upside down in the right inside breast pocket.

Note: a suit jacket is always called a coat.

WAISTCOATS

A traditional three-piece suit creates a distinguished look. A waistcoat lengthens the body and the continuation of suit fabric from neck to toe is flattering to all shapes. Some say they act a bit like a corset. Waistcoats should have six or seven buttons.

Note: the bottom button is left undone.

THE BRITISH SUIT

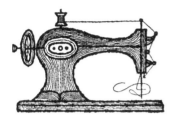

☞ A traditional British suit should be single-breasted, and usually single or double-buttoned. ☞ *The shoulders should be neither too narrow nor too wide. They are padded to provide structure rather than bulk.* ☞ There should also be a sharp, 90-degree angle between the shoulder and the sleeve of the suit. ☞ *The waist should show off your shape, with a slight flare over the hips.* ☞ The length of the coat (jacket) should be proportional to your height; it should reach the halfway point between the ground and the top of the coat's collar. ☞ *Traditionally, British suit coats feature side vents (rather than an American-style central vent) and slanted pockets.* ☞ British suits have a high gorge (the area where the lapel and the collar meet) meaning that less shirt is shown; the lapels should be a moderate width. ☞ *Trousers should rise to fit on the top of the pelvis. Flat-fronted trousers suit slim builds, but pleated trousers are usually more comfortable. Forward pleats that fold towards the fly are standard on Savile Row.* ☞ Trousers should break slightly at the front, but not at the back. As a general rule, turn-ups don't suit the line of a single-breasted suit.

TAILORS' TIPS: ☞ A tailor wants you to look your best, so trust his judgement. The suit your tailor wears advertises his style; if you don't like his suit then don't ask him to make you one. ☞ *Be honest. Don't suck in your stomach and push out your chest when being measured: the finished suit won't fit.* ☞ Tell your tailor where, how and when you will be wearing your suit. ☞ *Pocket space can be found for a phone, wallet or keys, so you should tell him what you usually carry around.* ☞ A good-quality suit should improve with age by moulding itself to your body.

TAILORS

Bespoke: a suit made completely from scratch. Every aspect, from fit, shape and style to the finer details, is tailored to the wearer.
Custom: fabrics, number of buttons, double or single-breasted, style of trousers etc can be chosen, but the cut of the suit will not change. Also known as semi-bespoke.
Bits Hand-Finished: an off-the-peg garment on which the cuffs and buttons are unfinished; the button height and sleeve length can therefore be altered.
Ready-to-Wear: designed to fit an average chest size and height. Sleeve lengths can be adjusted, waists can be taken in and general alterations can be made.

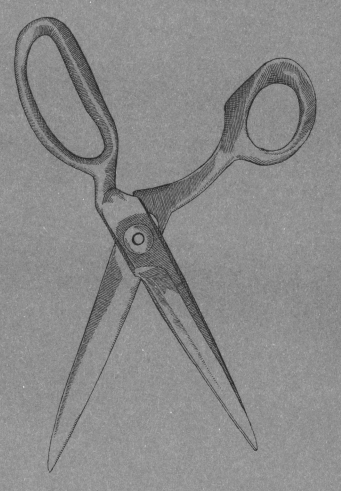

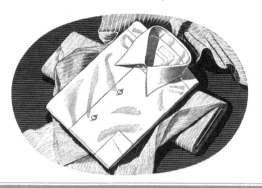

SHIRTS

A SHIRT THAT FITS: ☞ The fit of the yokes (the bit over the shoulder) is crucial to the fit of the shirt. ☞ *Shoulder pleats will allow for fullness in the back; a centre pleat is required for a slim fit.* ☞ Sleeves must be long enough to show some cuff when worn with a suit jacket. ☞ *The cuff (single or double with cufflinks) should end four and a half inches from the end of the thumb.* ☞ If you are an average build, opt for a close-fitting, flat front (the fullness should be in the back). ☞ *The tails should be long enough to ensure that they never pop out of the waistband.* ☞ You should be able to fit three fingers inside the collar at the side of the neck. ☞ *Avoid pockets on formal shirts – keep it simple and classic.*

FABRIC COUNTS

When it comes to cotton, the higher the number (thread count), the finer the fabric. Traditional business shirts are usually two-fold 140 or 120 weight cotton (two-fold 200 is the highest weight that is practical before it becomes too fine); soft, two-fold poplin is also a popular option.

GO BESPOKE

The benefits of a bespoke shirt are plentiful. It will actually fit you; it can be made to suit your needs; you can choose the best fabric; you can even choose the colour of the thread. With proper care, it may last for ten years. Moreover, tailors know what looks good so they can advise you on what suits you. Wearing clothes that are made for you can only increase your confidence and feel-good factor.

COLOUR COUNTS

Choose a coloured shirt carefully, first matching it to your skin tone and then thinking about the colour of your suits. Blue shirts are a safe choice, and white shirts generally go with everything – opt for a texture such as a herringbone twill to make it more interesting.

WASH WELL

Dry cleaning will wear out your shirts, particularly under the arms where deodorant will not be removed. It is, therefore, better to wash them at home after each wear. Remove the collar stays, undo the buttons and turn it inside out (to protect the buttons); a 40-degree wash is the usual option but check the care instructions. Iron when damp or take it to the dry cleaner for pressing.

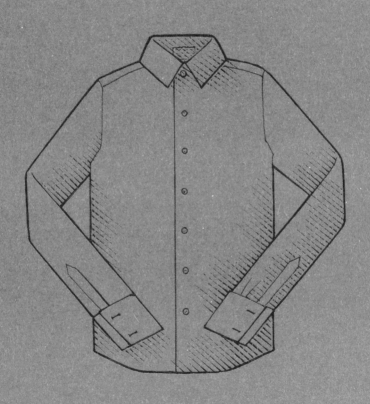

HOW TO IRON A SHIRT

Equipment: cotton shirt, iron, ironing board

METHOD:

☛ *Iron the underside of the collar first. Then, iron the outside, from the points to the centre, to avoid creasing the tips.*

☛ *Iron the cuffs, unbuttoned and with double cuffs unfolded. Start with the inside.*

☛ *Work from the top of the sleeve to the cuff. The addition of a crease is a matter of personal choice.*

☛ *Fit the shirt over the narrower end of the board and iron the yoke.*

☛ *Utilise the wide end of the board to iron the back.*

☛ *Lastly, iron the front panels, around the buttons. Pay special attention to the panel with the buttonholes, which will be on show when the shirt is worn.*

Top tip: the shirt should be damp (preferably from the wash) – never try to iron a dry shirt because the creases will not be removed effectively. The shirt and cuffs should be unbuttoned, and any collar stays removed.

Ironing rules: before you begin, always check the label and the fabric before setting the temperature on the iron. Never iron a dirty shirt and never iron over the buttons; use the tip of the iron to go round them. And don't forget to unplug the iron when you've finished.

Promises, promises: never buy a shirt whose label proclaims that is does not need ironing.

TIE RULES: ☛ Ties serve no practical purpose, so they may as well serve a sartorial one. ☛ *A tie's colour and pattern should complement your suit and shirt.* ☛ The best ties are made of silk, with a wool interlining. ☛ *The only knots you need are the four-in-hand and the half-Windsor.* ☛ Avoid garish Windsor knots that require a wide, cut away collar. ☛ *Never tuck your tie into your trousers; it should reach just above the waistband.* ☛ A tie, when worn with a suit, should always be properly done up. ☛ *Avoid ties that are too wide or too narrow.* ☛ Never wear a novelty tie.

TIES

FOUR-IN-HAND

This is the most basic tie knot. It is classic and discreet, ideal for a standard dress shirt. Start with the wide end of the tie hanging a foot below the narrow end. Bring the wide end up and through the hole at the neck, then thread it through the knot. Pull the knot up to the neck to tighten.

HALF-WINDSOR

Start with the wide end on the right, hanging a foot below the narrow end. Cross the wide end over the narrow, then back underneath. Bring the wide end up and then down through the loop. Bring the wide end across from left to right. Turn the wide end up, through the neck loop and through the knot in front.

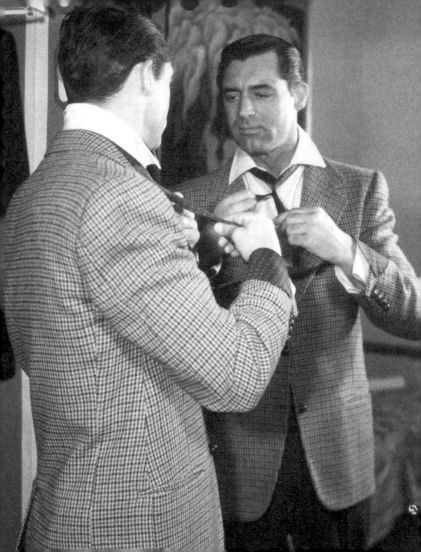

DRESS CODES COUNT

SPECIAL OCCASIONS require a multitude of different dress codes. For private events such as parties, balls etc, the dress code will usually be stated on the invitation. Public events – Royal Ascot, Henley Royal Regatta etc – vary in formality and the required dress code may depend on your ticket or enclosure badge. Dress codes should be strictly observed. Failure to comply would be considered rude or, at worse, you may be refused entry.

WHAT TO WEAR

JOB INTERVIEWS

First impressions really count, so try to interpret the office culture. If you're looking for your big break in the City, then don your very finest suit. In a more creative or less formal environment, stick to the classics but err on the smart side. Jeans are usually a touch too casual.

WEDDING DRESS

Wedding etiquette dictates that dress codes are not included on a wedding invitation unless there is an uncustomary code (such as black tie). If a dress code is stated, guests should take note and dress accordingly. Traditionally, wedding dress attire for men is morning dress, or a suit with a shirt and tie.

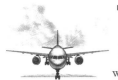

☛ **Aeroplanes:** always wear a collar, unless you're in cattle-class. ☛ *Bar Mitzvahs and Bat Mitzvahs: a formal suit and kippah.* ☛ **Bed:** solo winter nights = pyjamas; with company = boxers or *au naturel.* ☛ *Christenings: a suit and tie.* ☛ **Christmas:** no novelty jumpers. ☛ *Country House Opera: black tie is usually* de rigueur. ☛ **Dating:** dress for the occasion; be clean, smell good and look tidy. ☛ *Formal Dinners: double-check the invitation.* ☛ **Funerals:** a dark suit, a white shirt and a sombre tie. ☛ *Golf Club: check the clubhouse rules; jackets are often required.* ☛ **Gym:** sports shorts and t-shirt, always fresh and clean. ☛ *Henley Royal Regatta: Stewards' Enclosure: lounge suits, or rowing blazers or jackets and flannels, and a tie or cravat.* ☛ **Hollywood Black Tie:** a *laissez-faire* attitude will prevail. Always includes a suit and shirt. ☛ *Lounge Suit: a suit and tie.* ☛ **Members' Clubs:** check in advance whether a jacket and/or tie is required. ☛ *Pub: no jacket required.* ☛ **Royal Ascot:** Royal Enclosure = black or grey morning dress; Grandstand = suit, shirt and tie. ☛ *Shooting: traditional = tweed four-piece shooting suit, garish socks and stout boots or wellingtons. Modern = warm, breathable clothing and a waxed jacket (always green or brown).*

WHITE TIE or *'full evening dress'*

☛ Black single-breasted tail coat with silk lapels (unbuttoned).
☛ *Black matching trousers, with two lines of braid down each outside leg.* ☛ White marcella shirt, worn with a detachable wing collar, cufflinks and studs. ☛ *Thin white marcella bow-tie; always hand-tied.* ☛ White marcella evening waistcoat, double or single-breasted. ☛ *Black patent lace-up shoes, always scrupulously clean and shiny.* ☛ A black overcoat and white silk scarf can be worn.
☛ Nowadays it is not necessary to wear a top hat.

DRESS CODES

MORNING DRESS or *'formal day dress'*

☛ Black or grey morning coat, single-breasted with peaked lapels, curved front edges sloping back at the sides into long tails.
☛ *Trousers should be grey with a grey morning coat; grey and black striped with a black coat.* ☛ Plain white shirt with a stiff turned down collar, double cuffs and cufflinks. Pale blue or pink is also acceptable. ☛ *Black or silver tie, in heavy woven silk (a tie will look better than a cravat).* ☛ Waistcoat: grey under a black morning coat, buff under a grey coat. Coloured waistcoats can look garish; never wear a backless waistcoat. ☛ *Highly polished black lace-up shoes.* ☛ Top hat: grey felt or vintage black silk.

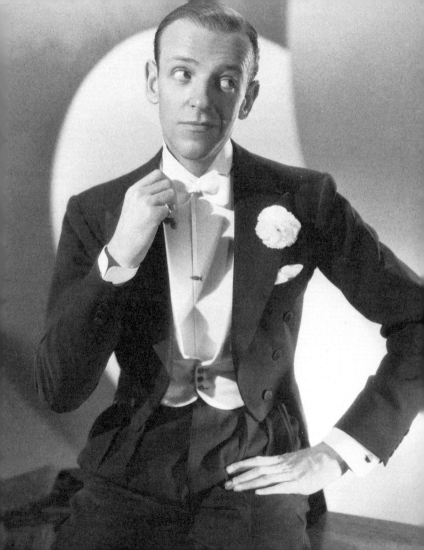

HOW TO TIE A BOW TIE

☛ Hang the tie around your neck, over the collar. ☛ *Adjust the tie so that one end is slightly longer than the other, crossing the long end over the short.* ☛ Bring the long end through the centre at the neck. ☛ *Form an angled loop with the short end of the tie crossing left.* ☛ Drop the long end at the neck over this horizontal loop. ☛ *Form a similar angled loop with the loose long end and push through the short loop.* ☛ Tighten by adjusting ends of both loops.

BLACK TIE

☛ **Black wool dinner jacket:** single-breasted with no vents, silk (often grosgrain) peaked lapels (or a shawl collar) and covered buttons. ☛ **Black trousers:** slightly tapered, with a single row of braid down the outside leg. ☛ **White marcella evening shirt:** soft turndown collar, worn with cufflinks and studs. ☛ **Bow tie:** always black, always hand-tied. ☛ **Lace-up shoes:** black, highly polished or patent. ☛ **Socks:** black silk, long enough to ensure that no leg will show when seated. ☛ **White silk scarf:** an optional, but traditional, accessory.

Note: Cummerbunds or black evening waistcoats are rarely worn nowadays.

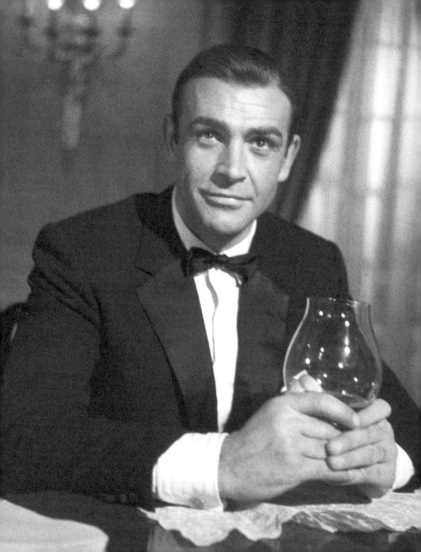

DECODING THE CODES

LOOK FOR THE LITTLE SIGNALS. The style of invitation and time of day is revealing, for example a printed invitation suggests a smarter event than a text or email, and an evening event is usually more formal than a daytime do. Whatever the occasion, smart casual requires a collar; never wear sportswear and always wear proper shoes. It's better to be overdressed than underdressed, and put a jacket in the car, just in case.

SMART CASUAL

CASUAL JACKETS

Jackets in a variety of materials, from linen and cashmere to tweed and pinstripe, can look stylish. Blazers are smart and formal, but keep your look sleek with a modern silhouette, slender lapels and non-metallic buttons. Pair either with jeans and a shirt and you'll be perfectly dressed-down.

CHINOS

Chinos provide a smart alternative to jeans, creating a relaxed yet traditional look. Go for a slim fit in a classic colour (khaki or navy, never red). For formal occasions, pair with a jacket, shirt and deck shoes; for a more casual look, wear with a polo shirt or casual shirt and plimsole-style shoes.

CASUAL SHIRTS

☛ Every wardrobe should have an Oxford shirt in blue and white. They look elegant and classic when paired with jeans, chinos and even shorts.

☛ Button-down collars should be buttoned.

☛ Choose classic patterns. Stripes can be flattering; checks should be small or gingham.

☛ Black shirts should be as dark and true-black as possible.

☛ Short-sleeved shirts are perfect for warmer days and mild evenings, but keep the fit slim over the arms.

☛ Wear the the shirt's collar button, and top one or two buttons, undone, depending on the distance between the buttons. Make sure you're not exposing too much chest.

☛ If you decide to wear a t-shirt underneath, choose the colour carefully.

KNITWEAR

☛ When paired with a shirt, a v-neck jumper will sit better than a round neck. Wear the collar on the inside.

☛ Wear plain, classic colours such as navy, black or grey.

☛ Avoid patterns, novelty motifs and intrusive branding.

☛ Go for a slim fit and avoid shapeless, baggy knits.

☛ Cardigans are perfect for layering, and for filling the gap when it's too hot for a jumper but you need something light for warmth.

☛ Keep it smart and fitted, and a cardigan can almost double up as a jacket.

☛ Polo necks and turtlenecks only suit a select few. Be wary.

FORMAL COATS: For timeless style, choose a CROMBIE. Thigh-length, single-breasted and occasionally with a velvet collar, this is the quintessential English town-coat. Similarly formal, a CHESTERFIELD is also thigh-length, double or single-breasted, woollen and often in grey herringbone. For a shorter option, a hip-length, double-breasted, navy PEA COAT is smart with a casual touch. This style, originally worn by sailors, will give you a *soupçon* of naval class.

NB: Formal coats should always be hung up properly and kept scupulously clean.

COATS

CASUAL COATS: The iconic navy, brown or black hooded DUFFEL COAT is a quirky choice – toggles are a must. Practical and hard-wearing, a PARKA has a warm fur-lined hood, and capacious body and pockets. For a lightweight coat, look no further than the classic waist-length, zip-fronted HARRINGTON.

WEATHER BEATERS: For proper protection, opt for a TRENCH COAT (worn collar-up) or a traditional MACKINTOSH (the original waterproof jacket). A WAX JACKET, once only seen in the countryside, is now a strikingly British staple. Usually in brown or green, it is an investment that will last you a lifetime.

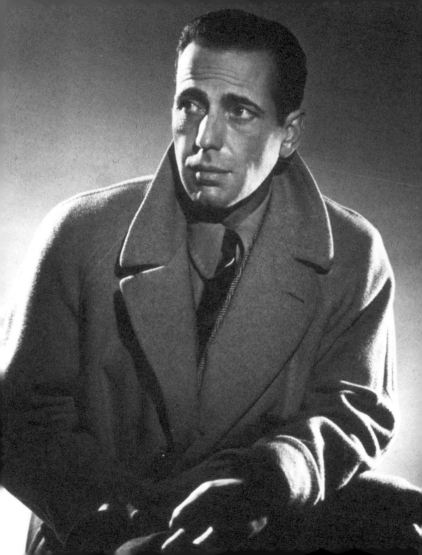

WELL-SHOD

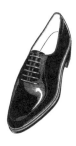

Your shoes say it all. A man is
frequently judged by his shoes so,
when it comes to getting dressed,
remember to think about your feet.
Shoes are a critical component of an
outfit – get ready to put your best
foot forward.

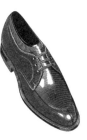

SHOES

FOOTWEAR ESSENTIALS: ☛ Formally, laces should be of the
same colour as the shoe. Informally, create an eye-catching look by
sporting brightly coloured ones. ☛ *Your soles should be made of
leather; avoid wearing them in the rain until they are worn in and
a little scuffed.* ☛ Your shoes will need to be taken to a cobbler if
there is a very soft spot in the sole at the front of the shoe, in the
middle, where the ball of your foot sits. ☛ *Never add stick-on soles
or metal clips to either the toes or the heels; these upset the balance
of your shoe and make a racket when you walk.*

BROGUES are the classic business shoe. Perfect with a suit, they can also be dressed down with jeans when in brown. Identified by the distinctive patterns across the toe, and available as a full or half-brogue, this is the essential shoe for every wardrobe.

The OXFORD is the epitome of English style – understated, classic and perfect with a suit. Similar in shape to a brogue, though without the patterned toes, they should be of black or brown polished leather; more casually they can also look good in suede.

Less formal than the Oxford or the brogue, though similar in shape, the DERBY shoe is simple and unfussy in either brown or black. Often with only two or three eyelets for lacing, they can dress down a suit or be worn casually with jeans.

LOAFERS are one of the most informal and convenient shoes, but wear with caution. An American innovation, developed by Italian shoemakers, they represent a Continental style and are best paired with chinos, jeans or shorts.

The ANKLE BOOT tends to look wrong with a formal suit and should, therefore, be avoided for smart dress codes. However, with slim fit suits, they can create a mod-like look which will work in less formal situations.

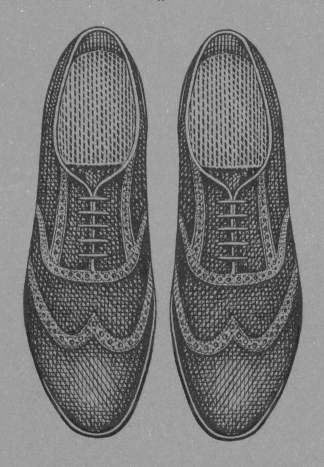

HOW TO POLISH SHOES

Equipment: leather shoes, newspaper, wax polish, cleaning cloth (damp), soft cloth (eg an old sock or t-shirt), polishing brush (preferably horsehair), duster

METHOD:

☞ *Protect the work surface with some newspaper.*

☞ *Remove shoelaces, but leave shoe-trees in.*

☞ *Clean off any loose dirt with a damp cloth.*

☞ *Wrap the soft cloth tightly around your first two fingers.*

☞ *Apply small amounts of polish all over the shoe in a circular motion.*

☞ *Leave for approximately 15 minutes, and then buff with the polishing brush.*

☞ *Finally, rub to a gleaming shine with a clean duster.*

Note: leather protector spray will help to maintain the shine.

Top tip: always put unvarnished cedar shoe-trees into your leather shoes as soon as you've removed them, while they are still warm, to help retain the shape and draw out any moisture. Leather shoes ought to be rested for a couple of days after they have been worn.

Shoe care S.O.S: if your shoes are wet, fill them with newspaper to absorb the moisture as they dry. Never leave them near a source of heat, like a fire or radiator, as this will instantly dry out the leather and warp the shape of the shoe.

HOW TO CHOOSE JEANS

☛ Try on lots of different styles and brands. ☛ *Every wardrobe should have three pairs of jeans: classic mid-blue, dark blue and black.* ☛ With a mid-rise waist and slim fit on the leg, a classic fit will suit most people. ☛ *Skinnier jeans suit shorter, slim legs. They should sit low on the waist and snugly hug the leg.* ☛ If you are of a bigger build then opt for a relaxed (but not too baggy) fit. ☛ *New jeans should fit around the waist and never need a belt.*

JEANS

WASHING: wear your new jeans for as long as possible before washing them (purists recommend six months), allowing them to mould to your body shape. Some say that the first wash should be at 60 degrees, without detergent. Subsequent washes should be on a cool, 30-degree cycle. Hang to dry; never tumble dry.

WEARING: there are very few occasions now where jeans are an absolute no-no. If your jeans are cut well and not looking too old and shabby, you will be suitably dressed in most situations. Smart jeans are becoming more acceptable in non-suit-wearing workplaces. Jeans with a suit jacket create a smart, yet dressed-down, look.

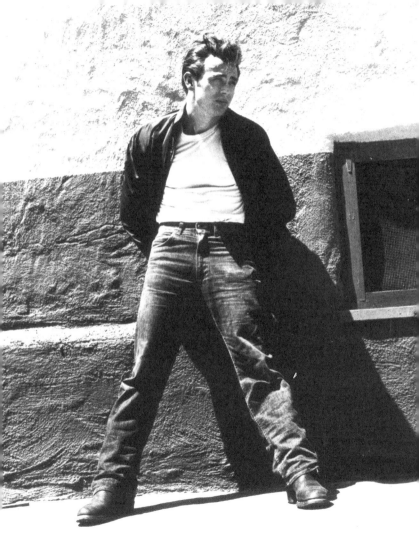

A WARDROBE STAPLE: ☞ Invest in a few good quality t-shirts that will endure regular wear and washing. ☞ *Opt for a slim fit, without it being too tight.* ☞ The sleeves should not dig into your biceps unless you've got a magnificent physique. ☞ *The length should fall slightly below the waist, but sit above the trouser pockets.* ☞ Plain colours are the most versatile; avoid logos, jokes and bold patterns. ☞ *Round-necks suit everyone; v-necks should be shallow and come well above the chest (hair).* ☞ White t-shirts should always be crisp and clean, without a hint of grey.

T·SHIRTS & POLOS

A TIMELESS CLASSIC: ☞ The polo shirt is a wardrobe essential – the collar creates a sense of formality that a t-shirt can't achieve. Keep it classic. ☞ *Experiment with different colours, stripes and trims. Don't be scared to go bold, especially during the hot summer months.* ☞ Opt for a slim fit (never go baggy), tailored to flatter the chest and upper back, that sits snugly around the upper-arm. ☞ *Opt for classic Piqué or soft jersey cotton.* ☞ Always wear untucked. ☞ *Logos and brand labels should be very discreet.*

Style Rule: band t-shirts are only acceptable if you attended that specific gig or if you own more than two of the band's records.

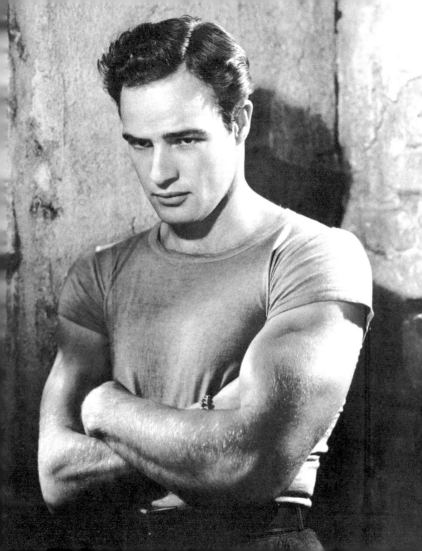

GYM ETIQUETTE

☛ Wipe down your equipment each time you use it. ☛ *Don't hog the machines.* ☛ Check your personal hygiene; no-one wants to smell you before they see you. ☛ *Mirrors are for honing your technique, not for self-admiration.* ☛ Music played through earphones should only be audible to you. ☛ *Keep noise to a minimum and refrain from grunting.* ☛ Don't get distracted by, or stare at, girls working out. ☛ Know your limits; don't overdo it.

SPORTSWEAR

ALL THE GEAR, NO IDEA

While the right kit is important, don't overdo it. There's no finer sight for a bowler than the batsmen bedecked in helmet, arm guard, chest guard and the latest bat, who can't play the simplest forward defensive. Likewise for any other sport: start with the basics, then move on from there.

ON THE PITCH

Though it won't hamper your performance, wearing a football shirt at a cricket match looks as wrong as whites on the rugby pitch. Also, a well turned out team will have an immediate advantage. It comes down to etiquette in the end; wearing the right kit is simply playing by the rules.

EXERCISE ESSENTIALS

☛ Before undertaking any exercise, ensure that your kit is fresh and clean. ☛ *Stay modest. You may be cooler in skimpier gear, but others won't want to be near you when you're lunging.* ☛ Start with shoes: there are different types for different forms of exercise and types of feet. Visit a specialist shop to get fitted properly but, generally, most people invest running and cross-training shoes. ☛ *Wear socks that cushion joints and absorb sweat.* ☛ Lightweight, sweat-free, and flexible, shorts are perfect for all forms of exercise. Avoid buttock-hugging Lycra unless they are worn under another pair of shorts. ☛ *Stretchy trousers are good for winter running. Tracksuit trousers are too heavy and will heat you up too quickly.* ☛ Vests should be made of a material that wicks sweat from the skin. ☛ *A jacket should be worn for winter running to keep out wind and rain. Reflective stripes help visibility, though not style.* ☛ A heart rate monitor is an essential piece of kit to determine your effort. Upgrade with a GPS monitoring device, micro-chipped shoes or phone apps for even better data.

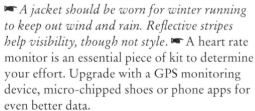

39

BEACH ETIQUETTE

☛ Never park too close to other people and maintain at least a towel's length between you and your neighbours. ☛ *Never steal someone else's sun, or hog the shade.* ☛ Shake towels with full consideration for wind direction. ☛ *If you must throw a ball, Frisbee or anything else around, do it as far away from anyone else as possible.* ☛ Never play music except through headphones. ☛ *Keep noise to a minimum.* ☛ Never (obviously) stare at girls.

AT THE BEACH

SAFE SUN

Protect yourself from the sun. Apply a broad spectrum, water resistant sunscreen (SPF 15 or higher) 30 minutes before you go out into the sun, and then every two hours. Remember, a tan offers no protection, so you must always wear sunscreen no matter how bronzed you are.

SAND STYLE

While you may be comfortable being half naked on the beach, it's no excuse to let standards drop – particularly when it comes to style. There are a surprising number of *faux pas* for an environment in which so few clothes are worn, so dress carefully and appropriately.

WHAT TO WEAR

☛TRUNKS that are slightly tailored, with a flat front and a straight slim fit, are surprisingly flattering. They also transfer from beach to bar with ease and style (*note: your trunks can double up as shorts; this also will prevent you from balancing on one foot under a towel trying to get changed*). ☛Alternatively, BOARD SHORTS provide a laidback, comfortable look and suit most people. TIGHT SHORTS should only be worn by those who are in tip-top shape. SKIMPY TRUNKS should never, ever be worn and it goes without saying that there is no place for MICRO-BRIEFS or THONGS (not even ironically). ☛Wear a hat: something straw usually looks good on sand. ☛A light cotton shirt, t-shirt or polo shirt is the best cover up and should always be worn when you are not on the beach, particularly in shops, bars and restaurants. ☛Choose your sunglasses carefully to suit your face – *follow the rules on pp. 42–43*. ☛Opt for easy footwear – flip-flops are the best choice but, if you have to cover any uneven ground before hitting the sand, wear canvas deck shoes (sports trainers never look good outside of the gym).

S UNGLASSES SHOULD BE AS WIDE AS YOUR FACE. Anything too big or too small will look out of proportion. The top of your frames should bisect your eyebrows, covering part of them but not all of them. Sunglasses should not ride up or slide down your nose; the bridge ought to be a snug, but not too tight, fit. They should feel comfortable over your ears and not pinch your temples, and your eyelashes shouldn't touch the lenses.

ROUND FACE =	SQUARE FACE =	OVAL FACE =
wide or rectangular frames	*oval or round frames*	*most frames will suit*

SUNGLASSES

CHECKLIST: ☛ Don't choose frames just to make a statement – they should suit both your face and style. ☛ *They should always offer proper UVA/UVB sun protection: check for certification.* ☛ Try before you buy. Don't buy online if you haven't already tried them on in a shop. ☛ *Avoid wearing sports sunglasses for casual wear; they won't suit non-sports clothes.* ☛ Stick to classic black, grey or amber lenses; avoid anything coloured or mirrored. ☛ *If you wear reading glasses, get some sunglasses with prescription lenses. Never double-up and wear two pairs of frames.* ☛ Avoid wearing your sunglasses inside – it's rarely sunny there...

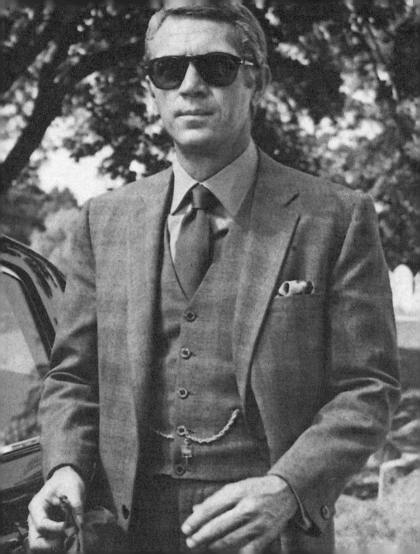

INVEST IN TIME

WATCHES ARE BECOMING less essential given the time-telling capabilities of modern portable devices. But a watch is never about just telling the time – it's the most important accessory in a man's wardrobe. It is both an investment and an heirloom, and, as a portable mechanical object, there is nothing better than a wristwatch. Having so many moving parts all working accurately on your wrist is precisely where the appeal lies.

WATCHES

WATCH CARE

Keep your watch away from water and only wear it when swimming or in the shower if it is water resistant to 100 metres. Extreme temperatures and magnetic fields may harm it; steer clear of detergents and solvents. Never over-wind the mechanism, and get it serviced every three to five years.

MULTIPLE CHOICE

If you're serious about your timepieces, start collecting. This will also give you the flexibility to match your watch to your outfit. There are certain watches that are wrong for certain occasions – for example, if you are wearing a dinner jacket, you don't want something too big and ostentatious on your wrist.

HOW TO BUY A WATCH

☛ A brand name should be a guarantee of quality. The more respected the brand, generally the better the watch. ☛ *Trust your instincts. You've been wearing a watch for most of your life, so you probably have a good idea of what you want.* ☛ Try on a lot of watches. What looks good in the shop or in an advert may not look good on your wrist. ☛ *It is false economy to spend money on watches that are built for short-term fashion.* ☛ Metal straps are generally longer-lasting than leather, but choose according to your style and desired look. ☛ *If you're buying a serious watch, you should be buying a mechanical one; look for heritage and long-term quality.* ☛ Indulge in the minutiae of the watch's movement, its mechanisms and details. Spend time in the shop asking questions and learning about it. ☛ *Watches are named after film stars and explorers for a reason. There's nothing wrong with feeling like one when you slip yours on.* ☛ Only buy a vintage timepiece from a reputable dealer; check that they can provide all the original documentation. ☛ *Choose carefully. Your watch should still retain its magic year after year.* ☛ Remember the money is in the craftsmanship of the mechanics and that they will outlast you.

UNDERWEAR BASICS

☞ There is no right or wrong type of underwear (except Y-fronts and thongs) – comfort is king. ☞ *Fitted underwear should be plain, not patterned, in white, navy, black or grey.* ☞ Never wear baggy boxers with a suit. ☞ *Your trousers should cover your underwear.* ☞ If wearing just boxers, remove your socks immediately. ☞ *Keep underwear clean. Your mother was right about that bus.* ☞ Going commando is for emergencies only.

ACCESSORIES

WEDDING RINGS

Once the preserve of women alone, it is now usual for married men to wear wedding bands – though it is certainly not compulsory. Choose a band that suits your hand, ensuring it is neither too wide and chunky nor too slim and feminine. Opt for gold or platinum; silver won't stand the test of time.

CUFFLINKS

Be very afraid of the novelty cufflink, but use cufflinks as a subtle expression of character – for example your love of cars may be revealed in driving-themed cufflinks. Enjoy the ritual of putting them on: once suited, shirted and shod, the fastening of cufflinks is a satisfying finishing touch.

ACCESSORY RULES

☛ Braces should always be button-on, rather than clip-on. ☛ *Pocket squares should be worn with a tie, but never match the tie.* ☛ Socks with suits should be discree and tactful, socks with jeans can be inventive. They must be long enough so when you sit down and cross your legs, you don't flash any calf-flesh. ☛ *A walking umbrella exudes style; a folding umbrella is more practical. A golf umbrella should never be seen away from the countryside.* ☛ Never wear mittens; gloves should be dark and cashmere. ☛ *Signet rings should be the real deal – no invented crests.* ☛ That necklace that looks great on the beach in the sunshine, works less well in the sleet in February. ☛ *Military-style dog tags should never be worn by a civilian.* ☛ Tie pins aren't necessary. ☛ *Key fobs should never advertise either the car you drive or the one you lust after.* ☛ Money clips are for those who feel the need to show off. ☛ *Leather belts should be black or brown (never shiny) with a discreet buckle. They should never be worn with a suit.* ☛ It takes a confident man to wear a hat; play it safe and keep it classic. ☛ *Scarves should be black or navy, and preferably cashmere.*

WALLETS: A BILLFOLD WALLET – the classic fold-in-half trouser-pocket wallet – is a practical option. Choose one for just cards or, more practically, go for one with a coin pouch. If you're after more of a formal, old-school look, a tall, slim COAT WALLET will fit inside your jacket pocket. Alternatively, A SLIMLINE WALLET provides room for essential cards. Their compact shape and size makes them a good option for suit-wearers. A LEATHER COIN PURSE stows cash safely – pockets of loose change will ruin your suit trousers.

BAGS & WALLETS

MAN BAG: The so-called 'man bag' is an accepted piece of everyday kit, and is essential for carrying around your MP3 player, keys, notebook, pen, PDA, tablet PC etc. A cross-body MESSENGER BAG is one of the most popular, practical and stylish options – it is casual enough to be worn at weekends, but functional enough to be a good choice for work. Alternatively, a plain RECORD BAG provides a casual and practical option. Either way, opt for subtle colour and minimal branding.

WORKBAGS

BRIEFCASES are classic, but they are not for everyone. Think about what will suit your style and your job. If you require a touch of formality, try a document bag with a leather shoulder/across-the-body strap. LAPTOP BAGS are, however, today's standard workbag. Choose one that suits your working wardrobe – leather is the stylish choice. Go for one with a strong buckle fastening and robust handles.

ON THE MOVE

Bigger than a standard wallet and designed to fit your passport, boarding pass, traveller's cheques and foreign currency, a TRAVEL WALLET is a must for the frequent-flyer. Those with zips are often the most secure and practical.

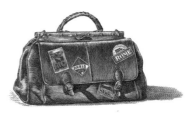

ESSENTIAL LUGGAGE

A SUIT BAG with added pockets is perfect for short hand-luggage-only trips away. A TROLLEY-BAG is useful when you need more than a suit bag, but less than a suitcase. Opt for one that can be carry-on luggage. Invest in a larger SUITCASE for longer holidays; durable, tough nylon is the most practical choice. A good-quality leather HOLDALL is invaluable for overnight stays or weekends away.

Etiquette tip: as a general rule, hotel bellboys or porters should be tipped one to two dollars, euro or pounds per case.

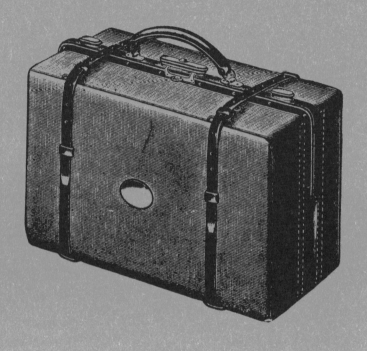

HOW TO PACK A SUITCASE

Equipment: suitcase, shoebags, tissue paper, shoes, clothes, washbag, accessories, jacket

METHOD:

☞ *Place shoes in the bottom. Roll socks and underwear; place inside shoes.*

☞ *Add the washbag; if using a trolley case, place at the wheel-end.*

☞ *Slot ties and belts into the spaces.*

☞ *Lay trousers flat across the case, leaving the legs hanging over the side.*

☞ *Fold shirts and place on top of the trousers.*

☞ *Carefully roll jumpers.*

☞ *Place your jacket on top. Fold in the sleeves to form a X.*

☞ *Draw up the overhanging trouser legs and wrap around everything.*

Be organised: pack the things you'll need first within easy reach – clean shirt, pyjamas, swimming trunks…

Be smooth: layer sheets of tissue paper among and on top of the clothes; hang creased shirts in a steamy bathroom.

Be protective: keep shoes in bags and make sure your toiletries are sealed tight.

Be clean: pack a small bag to keep dirty laundry separate, making it easy to sort your washing when you get home.

Be compact: keep it simple and don't overpack.

Be prepared: always pack an international adaptor plug and an umbrella.

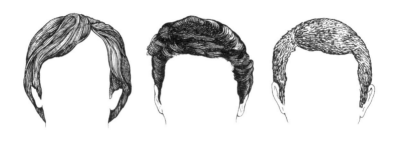

HAIR

BARBER ETIQUETTE

A T A TRADITIONAL WALK-IN BARBERSHOP, no one will be offended if you choose to wait for your favourite cutter to become free. Always be sociable and pleasant, and engage in small talk; your barber is experienced enough to distinguish the talkers from the thinkers, so don't feel obliged to hold conversation for the whole time if you don't want to. Don't use your phone to make or receive calls – it's rude to your barber and makes their job difficult. Always tip your barber around ten per cent. In salons, also leave a couple of pounds for the person who washed your hair.

HAIRSTYLES

As a general rule, men's hairstyles are short, medium or long. Your hair-type and face shape will determine much of what suits you, but your hairstyle should also be tailored towards your lifestyle.

Remember that your barber doesn't really know you so spend some time explaining what you want. Don't expect him to be a mind reader – you'll most likely come away disappointed. Equally, you must be realistic. Thinning or grey hair may not suit every style, so take his advice.

Aim to get your hair cut every five to six weeks – remember, unlike clothes, you wear your hair seven days a week, 24 hours a day, so it's worth the effort and the expense.

Short hair: maintain the style with a water-soluble matt paste; avoid heavy waxes.

Medium hair: add texture with a light, soft gel; avoid anything that will stiffen the hair.

Long hair: leave it to its own devices as much as possible; leave-in conditioner can tame fly-away tresses.

Receding hair: don't try to hide it – your barber can advise you on flattering styles.

Bald: accept the situation and shave it or keep it very short. Either way, it should be at a consistent length all over.

Grey: learn to love it. Approach dyes with caution – natural is best. Keep it short, regularly cut and well-styled.

HAIRY RULES

☛ Beards should be neither too manicured nor too wild. Use clippers to keep them neat and a consistent length. ☛ *A moustache can mask a large gap between the top lip and nose. Keep it tidy with a moustache comb.* ☛ If you have patchy growth or variations in colour, shave it off. ☛ *Facial hair should be kept scrupulously clean; wash regularly with shampoo.* ☛ Nurture your growth. Use hot flannels to steam the skin underneath, and moisturise regularly.

FACIAL HAIR

BEARD SHAPE

Draw an imaginary line from the top of your sideburn to the corner of your moustache: there should be no hair above this line. There should be no hair on your neck, just on the underside of your jaw above your Adam's apple. Pluck out any strays. A good beard requires regular maintenance.

EYEBROWS, EARS & NOSES

Avoid a mono-brow by plucking between your two brows. Never over-pluck or you risk looking startled. If in doubt, get it done by a professional. Nasal-hair trimmers are a cheap, effective and essential piece of gear. Use them. And don't forget about your ears.

54

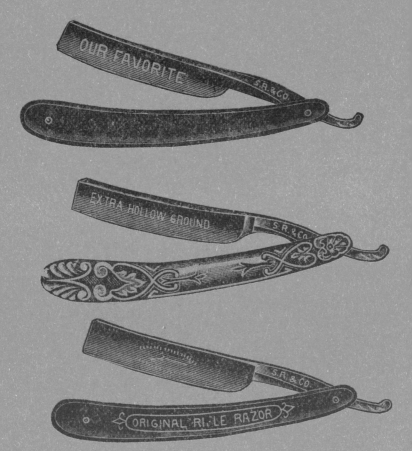

HOW TO SHAVE

Equipment: hot and cold water, flannel, shaving cream or soap, brush, multi-blade razor, stubble

METHOD:

☞ *Hold a hot flannel to your face to open up your pores.*

☞ *Using a circular motion, apply shaving cream or soap.*

☞ *Shave in the direction of the hair growth; this changes on different parts of the face, and especially on the neck.*

☞ *For a very close shave, hold another hot flannel on your face to reopen your pores.*

☞ *Brush on another application of shaving cream or soap, and shave in the opposite direction to which the hair grows.*

☞ *Once finished, hold a cold flannel against your face to close up your pores.*

☞ *Use a moisturiser, shaving balm or aftershave gel asap.*

Cut-throat in the Chair

A cut-throat shave is done at the barbers, and is not advised for those who use electric shavers (the skin will not be conditioned). After some hot towels and an application of soap, the barber shaves with the grain of the beard, in as few strokes as possible, before then shaving against the grain. The shave is finished with an application of a cold towel, shaving balm and aftershave.

Shaving cuts: use a styptic pencil dipped in water.

Razor rash: rub an alum block, dipped in water, on your face to reduce redness and irritation.

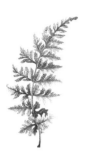
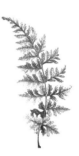

STYLISH SCENT

Citrus *fresh and energising*
Aromatic *lavender and herbal*
Aquatic *cooling and maritime*
Fougère *woody and mossy*
Chypre *leathery yet fresh*
Oriental *incense and spices*

AFTERSHAVE

A FRAGRANCE'S TRUE SMELL takes a while to develop. After that initial spray, you are hit with the citrus and top notes – fresh and fruity, they are a stimulating welcome to the scent. After about 20 minutes, the flowery, spicy and woody aromas of the heart notes start to take shape. Essentially, this is what your fragrance will smell like for most of the time. The remainder are known as the base notes. Vanilla, musky, woody or smoky, these are the smells that are noticeable on your clothes after you've worn a fragrance.

FRAGRANCE ESSENTIALS

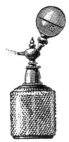

☞ When buying a fragrance, try just a few at a time to avoid a confusing sensory overload. Leave it at least 20 minutes for the true aromas to develop. ☞ *Consider the weather. While it is appealing to have a 'signature' scent, some smells are better suited to the heat of summer, while others suit the colder winter months.* ☞ Think about when you will be wearing it. One fragrance may not comfortably work for both the office and evenings out. ☞ *Apply fragrance to your pulse points, such as your wrist and neck. Also spray a few squirts onto your chest after a warm shower.* ☞ The longer you wear an aftershave, the less it seems to smell. Avoid upping the quantities or you risk overpowering those around you. It smells just as it always did – you're just used to it. ☞ *Eau de toilette is stronger than an aftershave, so limit yourself to two or three squirts on the chest and pulse points, but check that you're not overdoing it.* ☞ Fragrance should be stored in a cool, dark place. Avoid the bathroom because of temperature fluctuations; keep the bottle in its box out of direct sunlight. ☞ *Your fragrance should complement your personality, style and the occasion.*

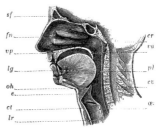

WASHING CLOTHES

☞ Separate darks, colours, whites etc. ☞ *Empty pockets; zip up zips.* ☞ Take note of garments' care labels. ☞ *Never wash anything at a higher temperature than stated on the label.* ☞ Turn patterned, printed or coloured items inside out before washing. ☞ *Use a mesh bag to protect delicate garments.* ☞ Don't overload the machine. ☞ *Don't use too much detergent or softener.* ☞ Empty the machine as soon as possible when its finished. ☞ *Never use bleach.*

CLOTHING CARE

CASHMERE CARE

☞ Cashmere should be hand-washed in lukewarm water with a mild shampoo. ☞ *Rinse out in lukewarm water until it is clear.* ☞ Gently squeeze (never wring) the garment in a towel to remove excess water, and then dry flat away from direct light. Reshape while damp. ☞ *Pilling – tiny balls of fluff that are naturally caused by wear – can be removed with a special cashmere comb.* ☞ Store garments in breathable plastic bags; freshly laundered garments should be put away for the summer months.

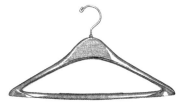

STORING CLOTHES

☞ Don't overload the hanging rail; clothes need plenty of room to breathe.

☞ Use suitably shaped wooden hangers (never wire).

☞ Empty pockets before you hang anything up.

☞ Jackets should be hung unbuttoned.

☞ Trousers should be hung unbuttoned and unzipped.

☞ Fold jumpers; hanging can pull them out of shape.

☞ Only put away clothes when they are completely dry.

☞ Rarely worn garments should be put away clean and protected with covers, or stored in bags.

LEATHER CARE

☞ Leather must be allowed to breathe, so never store it in plastic bags or non-porous containers.

☞ Spray items with a protector – avoid any products containing silicone or wax – and use leather conditioner to prevent it from drying out or cracking.

☞ Stuff leather bags with tissue to maintain their shape, and store in original dustbags.

☞ Hang leather jackets on wide or padded hangers.

☞ Use unvarnished cedar shoe trees in leather shoes.

☞ Air leather goods every couple of weeks to reduce the chance of mould.

☞ Always clean leather before you store it.

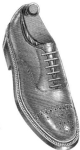

MEN'S STYLE A-Z

A ☞ **ACCESSORIES** should be classic and understated, never ostentatious and flashy. B ☞ **BESPOKE** tailoring will provide you with the finest garments – indulge in it if you can afford to do so. C ☞ **COATS** should always complement and coordinate with what you are wearing. D ☞ **DRESS CODES** should always be adhered to. It is better to be overdressed than underdressed. E ☞ **EXPERIMENT** with your style until you find one you're comfortable and confident with. F ☞ **FRAGRANCE** should complement your personality, style and the occasion. G ☞ **GYM KIT** should be modest, never skimpy. H ☞ **HAIR** should be well maintained; you wear it seven days a week, 24 hours a day. I ☞ **IRON** Shirts should always be freshly laundered and completely crease-free. J ☞ **JACKETS** are a wardrobe essential, pair with jeans for a perfect dressed-down look. K ☞ **KNITWEAR** should be plain, in classic colours such as navy, black or grey. L ☞ **LOUNGE SUITS** are normal business suits, worn in semi-formal situations with a shirt and tie. M ☞ **MOUSTACHES** and beards should be kept clean, neat and tidy. N ☞ **NOVELTY JUMPERS**, ties and socks may cause offence or dismay, even if the intention is ironic. O ☞ **OFFICE WEAR** differs from company to company; establish the prevailing style when you go for the interview. P ☞ **POLO SHIRTS** offer a more formal alternative to t-shirts. Q ☞ **QUALITY** clothes are worth the extra cash; they will withstand regular wear and washing. R ☞ ROUND-NECKED jumpers and t-shirts suit everyone; v-necks are less versatile. S ☞ SAVILE ROW is the home of British tailoring – explore its unique heritage. T ☞ TIE colour and pattern should complement your suit and shirt. U ☞ UNDERWEAR should never be on show when wearing trousers. V ☞ V-NECK JUMPERS are more suited to shirts than round neck jumpers. W ☞ WATCH An investment and an heirloom – the most important accessory in a man's wardrobe. X ☞ XL Sizing is important. Be honest with yourself and wear clothes that fit. Y ☞ Y-FRONTS and thongs are always wrong. Z ☞ ZZZZZ The End!

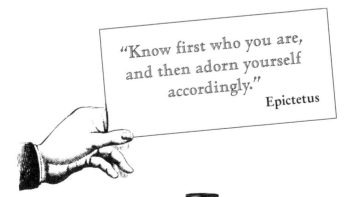

"Know first who you are, and then adorn yourself accordingly."

Epictetus

Also published by DEBRETT'S

Correct Form
Wedding Guide
Etiquette for Girls
Guide for the Modern Gentleman
Manners for Men
A-Z of Modern Manners
A Modern Royal Marriage
The Queen: the Diamond Jubilee

POCKET BOOKS:
Debrett's Netiquette

Debrett's also publishes an annual
range of stylish leather Lady's and
Gentleman's Diaries, with a wealth
of content that is designed to inspire,
inform and entertain.

Visit us at
www.debretts.com/shop

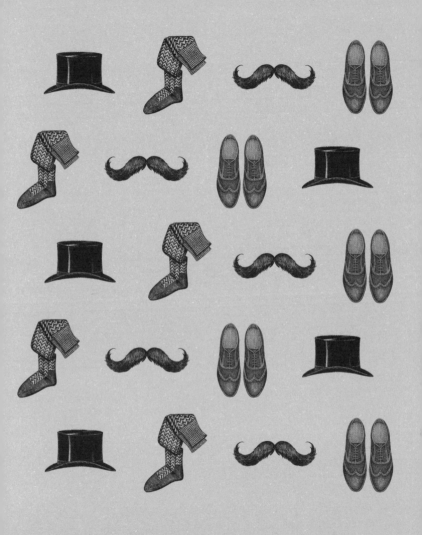